The Little Book Of
HOPE

Also by Joan McDonell

Half Crazy (a novel)

The Little Book Of
HOPE

Collected Writings on Depression, Despair & Melancholy

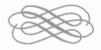

Compiled by
JOAN McDONELL

New Millennium Press
Beverly Hills

Library of Congress Cataloging-in-Publication Data

The little book of hope : compiled by Joan McDonell.
   p. cm.
  Includes bibliographical references and index.
  ISBN 1-893224-15-5 (hardcover)
   1. Depression, Mental—Quotations, maxims, etc. 2. Despair—Quotations, maxims, etc.
  3. Melancholy—Quotations, maxims, etc. I. McDonell, J. M.

RC537 .087 2001
616.85'27—dc21

                                                          00-033954

Printed in the United States of America

New Millennium Press
a division of NMWorldMedia, Inc.
301 N. Canon Drive
Suite 214
Beverly Hills, California 90210

10 9 8 7 6 5 4 3 2 1

For Terry

We do not see
things as they are,
we see things
as we are.

The Talmud

CONTENTS

FOREWORD

Nothing helps one to understand as much as to be understood. When the veil of depression draws over our eyes, we often do not know what is happening. Depression occurs subtly. The changes in our perception of life and of those around us are insidious—so insidious, in fact, that we believe our increasingly despairing view of life is reality. In a way, it *is* reality. It is *our* reality. That reality is painful, so painful that those who have not experienced it do not believe we hurt as we do. Sometimes, when we seek help for the pain, we are told it is "all in our head" or "it is not real pain." This only adds to our hopelessness and depression. No one understands. And what is worse, people seem not to care because the pain is "not real." We do not have cancer or AIDS. We are not paraplegic. Many of us are quite healthy. Some are young, or rich, or good-looking. In some instances we may be all. But we still hurt. Despairing of relief and in need of understanding, we want to die, and some of us do . . . by our own hand.

Joan McDonell, in this well-wrought volume, provides comfort for those who are suffering the pain of depression. Many of the quotes here are from people who have felt the sting and experienced hellish despair themselves. They are able to provide the kind of insight that even the most sensitive psychiatrist, if he or she has not suffered from depression, cannot.

The worst aspect of depression is, no doubt, the sense of hopelessness we feel; the certainty that things will never improve, will only get worse. Degree of hopelessness, unfortunately, is our best predictor of suicide. There are, however, many reasons to be hopeful at this turn of the new century. Now that depression is acknowledged to be as real as high blood pressure, we have much more support and many more resources; we also have a wider range of medication than ever before.

There are genetic (depression runs in families) and biochemical factors that interact with psychological and social forces to create depression and produce almost an expectation of future despair. Our genes determine changes in chemicals in the brain that have an impact on feelings and behavior. These chemicals—called neurotransmitters because they cause connections between nerve cells—include serotonin, dopamine, and norepinephrine. Serotonin, dopamine, and norepinephrine are amines. A deficiency of amines in the brain causes depression.

There is an ironic twist to our understanding of depression and suicide. Just as the fire given by Prometheus to man has stoked the fire that consumed victims of the Inquisition or entire villages in war, so too has it provided energy for the creation of the industrial era, which liberated man from the wild forces of nature. Depression comparably has not only caused much pain, but also, as this book reveals, directed the energy of many afflicted with it to create the artistic, political, and entrepreneurial achievements of which we are so proud and which have comforted the souls of many not afflicted with the pain. The poet Thomas Moore (1779–1852) stated: "The heart that is soonest awake to the flowers is always the first to be touched by the thorns." Vincent van Gogh, Sir Winston Churchill, and many others whose words are included in this book were driven to create a world as they would have liked it to be rather than as they often felt it.

The challenge to psychiatrists treating those with mood disorders is to assuage pain, redirect the emotional forces tearing at the soul, and create new ways to empower talent and strength—giving hope not only to the depressed person, but also to those who have suffered with him and because of him.

In the pages that follow, you may, as I did, find yourself stopping after a passage and reflecting. How beautiful the words. How deeply the pain felt. Would it ever have been possible for some of those represented in this book to achieve what they did without pain? I doubt it. Is it possible to experience the warmth of a midsummer breeze in the night without also experiencing the bitter cold of an arctic front that envelops all in its wake? I certainly believe it is.

Andrew E. Slaby, M.D., Ph.D.
Clinical Professor of Psychiatry
New York University
New York Medical College
March 2000

PREFACE

THE FIRST WORK excerpted in this book that I remember reading is the poem "Richard Cory" by Edwin Arlington Robinson, and that was thirty years ago. Since then, having read many novels, letters, poems, journals, biographies, articles, and graffiti, I realized that from the present all the way back thousands of years to the beginning of recorded history, people have been communicating their despair and melancholy. What I find most fascinating is that everybody has used and continues to use almost exactly the same ideas and words to describe these feelings.

Each and every person, from each and every period since the beginning of the written word, describes the symptoms of depression in much the same way. Certain usage of language and labels has changed, but the meaning remains completely consistent.

This collection represents my own personal and quite certainly erratic readings and fragments, pieces, and snippets saved over many years. There are enormous gaps, of course, and no doubt errors. Worst of all, there are missing attributions and biographical material, and not because I didn't look. For whatever is missing, misquoted, or incorrect, I apologize in advance.

The following passage by Giacomo Leopardi—although perhaps not easy reading—is one explanation of why I gathered all these pieces. Leopardi, a nineteenth-century Italian writer, was trying to describe works with universal applications, works of brilliance. Certainly there are geniuses—Shakespeare, Milton, van Gogh—represented in the collection, but it is my hope that the smaller stars also generate enough heat to help take the edge off the long, lonely, freezing nights of despair that many of us, great souls and regular souls and impoverished souls alike, endure. This is what Leopardi wrote

> Works of genius have this in common, that even when they vividly capture the nothingness of life, and when they express the most terrible despair, nonetheless to a great soul—though he find himself in a state of extreme duress, disillusion, nothingness, *noia*, and despair of life, or in the bitterest and dead-

liest misfortunes (caused by deep feelings or whatever)—these works always console and rekindle enthusiasms and though they treat or represent only death, they give back to him, at least temporarily, that life which he had lost.

So, dear reader, it is my sincerest hope that the words contained in the following pages will help console you and rekindle your enthusiasm for life most precious.

Joan McDonell
Amagansett, New York
May 2000

INTRODUCTION

THIS COLLECTION is for those of us who can see the light at the end of the tunnel but are sure—as the poet Robert Lowell said—that it's the light of an oncoming train. Or for others of us who are in the tunnel with no light at all. It's for people who are or have been in despair.

The history of despair, depression, and melancholy starts at the beginning of time. Despair almost always brings with it hopelessness and loneliness, and if that weren't bad enough, trying to explain despair to another person is very difficult. Few understand, and when you are nearly paralyzed by depression, you probably wonder, "Why bother?" because a depressed person usually thinks with the same certainty about pure despair as about pure love: it will never end.

Depression makes us tired and weak, but if you have the strength to look through this collection, you'll see that all the entries—from the famous, the forgotten, and the anonymous—send a single message: In spite of our stubborn ideas to the contrary, we have many companions. Many people have felt just as tired, as weak, as lonely, as helpless, and as hopeless as we have—throughout all recorded time.

Some words of heed: To those clinging to the belief that their relatives, friends, and colleagues who suffer from depression can simply shake off the mood in any number of quick-fix ways—for example, by pulling themselves up by those proverbial and infernal bootstraps (bootstraps, by the way, as antiquated in fact as the idea they represent)—this book is not for you.

It is for us. Because those of us who endure depression suffer from a particularly vicious illness that destroys our vitality—robbing us of mental and physical energy, of enjoyment, clarity, desire, and hope. Depression also can destroy our good judgment. The psychological torment can be so unbearable, we sometimes believe only death can end it. We think, irrationally, that the ones we love would be better off without us. Some of us consider suicide; some of us go through with it.

Here is one thing I know for certain: People who commit suicide do not want to die. They simply want to end the pain. Nevertheless, suicide is, in fact, the eighth leading cause of death in the United States—the third leading cause of death among people ages fifteen to twenty-four. With the exception of the terminally ill, who act to stop their physical suffering as well as their mental anguish, people commit suicide because they are desperately depressed. The pain is so staggering that even an experienced New York psychiatrist told me he was shocked to hear elderly Holocaust survivors insist that suffering from depression was worse than enduring the misery of the death camps in World War II. Unlike the severely depressed, the Holocaust victims who survived clung to hope and knew, even as they watched their numbers decrease horrifically, they were not entirely alone.

Human beings are designed to attempt, at least, to stay alive. We've all heard the remarkable stories of survival against unimaginable odds. If we want to understand the survival instinct, we must try to understand the human spirit, which remains remarkably mysterious. We know for sure that it is supremely powerful. Yet we must remember that the human spirit can be terribly fragile as well: it can bend, warp, break, and die. We celebrate gargantuan feats of the heart and mind—but we as a culture have little sympathy or even patience for the sick spirit. We do not question the fact that a person with diabetes can die if deprived of insulin. We applaud the billions of dollars spent searching for a cure for cancer. To the victims of these illnesses, we give nothing but kindness. Yet although depression can kill as viciously as cancer, we seem to have little but contempt, anger, and fear with regard to the depressed. Insulin and chemotherapy are never questioned, whereas lithium, even today in the twenty-first century, marks one as a crazy person and a pariah.

Statistics on mental illness differ, largely because much goes unreported. The U.S. Surgeon General and research published in the top medical journals estimate that 25 million Americans suffer from depression. According to the World Health Organization (WHO), this sickness costs U.S. employees $53 billion a year due to absenteeism and diminished productivity. WHO has predicted that by the year 2020, depression will be the leading cause of disability in developing countries. Further, in December 1999, the U.S. Attorney General announced that one out of two Americans can expect to suffer from some type of mental illness over the course of a lifetime.

The unspeakable pain of depression and the tragedy of suicide can be eliminated only by treating the illness. Unfortunately and frustratingly, the treatment—neither a science nor an art—remains elusive. There is no customary way to measure this affliction: no fever, no broken bones, no unusual heart rate or blood levels, nothing that shows up on MRIs, sonograms, or CT scans. Depression can be brought on by a situation, or it can follow a purely physical illness, but sometimes it appears without explanation. Some people have one episode; others are chronically depressed. Depression is an equal opportunity destroyer, striking all ages, from children to the elderly, and ignoring all gender and socioeconomic distinctions. It appears to run in families—but not always.

Until about ten years ago, there was no drug created specifically for depression. Before that— but not more than fifty years before, when there were no drugs at all—medicines were discovered by mistake; for example, while testing Elavil for use in combating tuberculosis, researchers noticed that one of the control groups seemed rather cheerful.

Today a variety of drugs, most famously Prozac, are available, but the type, combination, and dosage of medication represent little more than the best kind of informed guessing by even the most sophisticated psychopharmacologists. Faced with virtually no other choice, a program of psychotropic drugs and traditional talk therapy is the correct decision for almost any patient. The majority of people are not aware that electroshock treatment, which can be quite effective in extreme cases of depression, is no longer anything like it was in the past—most notably as depicted (negatively) in the 1975 film *One Flew over the Cuckoo's Nest*. In spite of enormous advances, many still find the very word *electroshock* terrifying. Alternative methods such as acupuncture, herbs, meditation, hypnosis, and changes in diet and exercise may indeed be useful in the treatment of depression, but to date no sufficiently thorough documentation exists.

Often those who suffer from depression don't know what caused the horrible darkness to descend. Whatever issue might have precipitated the illness (although depression is not always necessarily brought on by an event), however, brain chemistry is always involved. Exotic-sounding chemicals, hormones, and neurotransmitters such as norepinephrine, cortisol, and the much-publicized serotonin are the culprits and the saviors.

Those who are depressed often do not wish to talk about it, knowing too well that a fairly heavy stigma is still attached to this problem and wanting to avoid the additional burden of being considered crazy. The sufferer tries to hide the illness, and this hiding can become (to borrow a term from the self-help universe) denial.

Discussion of the illness is especially hard on men, since it challenges the still tightly held idea of masculine strength. For men, suffering is OK if you break a leg skiing, if you get a headache from sitting in front of the computer, or if your wife or girlfriend walks out on you. It's not OK, though, to have "sadness for no reason"—as the writer Tom McGuane once put it.

One man whose own despair has been chronicled quite extensively is Sir Winston Churchill, who gave many brilliant speeches, one of which contained the vividly remembered, often-quoted phrase: "There is one cardinal rule for the English nation . . . Never Despair." Of course, those close to Churchill knew about his lifelong battle with depression, but almost none of the English public was aware of it until after his death.

Depression is insidious. It can seep into one's consciousness after a loss or even a perceived loss—of work, of money, of love, of youth. It often follows a heart attack or a viral illness, like the flu. It can team up with hormonal changes to torture women—who suffer twice as much from depression as men and *report* many more cases than do men. Depression can accompany the diminution of light, creating a subaffliction known as seasonal affective disorder. It can also cast its oppressive shadow for no discernible reason at all.

The depressed person sometimes finds others to be sympathetic—but only up to a point. After a while, friends and family usually get confused, frustrated, uneasy, or irritated. Those not so close drop away. A depressed person is *not* fun to be with. Sometimes he gets angry, or blames others for his unhappiness, or (to use another psychological buzzword) "self-medicates" by drinking or taking drugs or overeating—or maybe he eats nothing. To add to his own confusion and the confusion and frustration of those around him, a clinically depressed person can go through the motions of daily life: he can go to work, go shopping, and go out to dinner. It's no wonder that most people find it nearly impossible to understand how a person who ordinarily looks fine and who continues on his daily rounds could be suffering from utterly debilitating psychic pain. All too often, this treacherous and paralyzing illness destroys not only its specific victims but also their families, friendships, careers, and marriages. Bruised and beaten by the proximity of an almost palpable despair, many decent people give up on and desert the suffering individual, the source and explanation of whose misery is so mysterious.

Many well-known people—Barbara Bush, Boris Yeltsin, Tipper Gore, Harrison Ford, and Dolly Parton among them—have spoken publicly of their own battles with depression. Each acknowledgment helps further the public's general enlightenment. Such well-known people, however, get a special break—not with their illness, but with the *perception* of their illness. Because they are so frequently seen looking and acting perfectly well,

they are not stigmatized and punished for their illness. Nonetheless, they are brave and generous to come forward into a society that not so terribly long ago forced Senator Thomas Eagleton out of the vice-presidential race when he revealed he had once received electroshock treatments for depression.

Ten years ago, who could have imagined that hand transplants or cloning would be possible beyond the realm of speculative fiction? We continually see astonishing progress affecting so many areas of medicine—except in the area of mood disorders. In his book *Darkness Visible*, William Styron recounted a conversation with a clinician in the field of depression. The clinician said, "If you compare our knowledge with Columbus's discovery of America, America is still unknown." Not much has changed between 1990, when the book was first published, and today.

Researchers are constantly at work on new medications. And the right medication does have a positive effect. But what *is* the right medication? Like the illness itself, the medicine is, at the least, exasperating. Unlike most medical problems, in which the physician simply treats the patient, depression requires an unusually strong partnership between patient and doctor. Because one of the symptoms of the disease is the powerful feeling that *nothing* can help, securing the patient's commitment to finding the right drug or combination of drugs is terribly difficult.

There is nothing easy about battling this affliction, but we have no choice. In combination with medication, talk therapy, available in many formats, is very helpful, if not crucial. Finding the right therapist can be as enervating as finding the right drug. For one thing, a psychopharmacologist—a physician versed in brain chemistry and the treatment of mood disorders—is not always the right person to see for talk therapy. The psychopharmacologist may not offer therapy, or he or she may not be right for you. Exercise also has a positive effect on almost anybody who suffers from depression. But when all one's strength is required just to get out of bed in the morning, it's hard to imagine a regular routine of rigorous exercise.

So there's a lot of bad news when it comes to depression. To avoid it, many of us who suffer from this illness become very good actors. We don't mention our depression because we've found that discussing it at best puts people off, and at worst puts our jobs—and our livelihoods—at risk. A result of this silence is that we don't know one another.

We read regularly—and the Surgeon General's report confirms—that one in ten Americans, 25 million people, suffer from depression. But where are they? Doctors and journalists indicated that no report from the Surgeon General's office since the 1964 report on smoking has been so important as this one. Was anyone paying attention? Who are those people who anonymously logged on to the National Depression and Manic Depression home page on the Internet during those first three sunny weeks of July 1999? Nobody knows, because we don't talk about it and they don't either. We don't know that our lawyer, our next-door neighbor, the woman behind the counter at the dry cleaners, the tennis coach, the man who sells tires, and the doctor in the emergency room are all as profoundly sad as we are. They are feeling just as isolated and just as hopeless. The most terrible and debilitating symptoms, again, are the feelings of hopelessness and loneliness.

We must remember that depression is a mood disorder, not a mood. It's a treatable illness, not a character flaw. It's not contagious like the flu, but it's been around forever. Remarkably, nothing has changed about the feelings of despair since the beginning of time. Whether by happenstance or deliberately, some of those who suffered left messages for us. In the following pages, people from different centuries and different cultures express the identical feelings of sadness and isolation—pointing out to us, of course, that we are not now, and never have been, alone.

COLLECTED
WRITINGS

Some are born to
sweet delight

Some are born to
endless night.

William Blake
"Augeries of Innocence," 1863

If there
is hell
upon earth,
it is to be found
in a melancholy
man's heart.

Robert Burton
The Anatomy of Melancholy,
1621

One may have a blazing hearth in one's soul and yet no one ever comes to sit by it.

Vincent van Gogh
Letter to his brother, Theo

I can't read or sleep. Without hope or youth or money I sit constantly wishing I was dead.

Zelda Fitzgerald
Letter to her husband,
F. Scott Fitzgerald

It is such
a secret place,
the land of tears.

Antoine de Saint-Exupéry
The Little Prince, *1943*

I am alone,
I am bereft, and the
night falls upon me.

Victor Hugo
"Booz endormi" (Boaz Asleep),
La Légende des siècles, *1883*

Suicides have a special language.
Like carpenters they want to
know which tools.
They never ask why build.

Anne Sexton
"Wanting to Die," 1966

Lay in the sun far up the beach, but the sun was cold, and the wind colder. The boom boom of great guns in my throat, then the ride back, bad tempered.

Sylvia Plath
1957
Published in The Journals of Sylvia Plath, *1982*

There is no vulture
like despair.

Marquis of Lansdowne

Mysteriously and in ways that are totally remote from natural experience, the gray drizzle of horror induced by depression takes on the quality of physical pain.

William Styron
Darkness Visible, *1990*

With nothing to look
back on with pride

And nothing to look
forward to with hope.

Robert Frost
"Death of a Hired Man,"
North of Boston, *1914*

There is never any logical reason for despair. . . You can't reason yourself into cheerfulness anymore than you can reason yourself another six inches in height.

Stephen Fry
1996

Sadness is more
like a head cold—
with patience
it passes.
Depression
is like cancer.

Barbara Kingsolver

I cannot remember the
time when I have not
longed for death . . . for
years and years I used to
watch for death as no sick
man ever watched for
morning.

Florence Nightingale
Quoted in Florence
Nightingale *by Cecil*
Wordham-Smith

The sad
companion,
dull-eyed
melancholy.

William Shakespeare
Pericles, *1609*

There seems to be so
much more winter than
we need this year.

Kathleen Norris
Bread into Roses, *1936*

In the country of
pain, we are each
alone.

May Sarton

I am now experiencing myself all the things that as a third party I have witnessed going on in my patients— days when I slink about depressed.

Sigmund Freud

I am now the most miserable man living. If what I feel were equally distributed to the whole human family, there would be not one cheerful face on earth. Whether I shall ever be better, I cannot tell. I forebode I shall not. To remain as I am is impossible. I must die or be better it appears to me.

Abraham Lincoln
Letter to John T. Stuart
January 23, 1841

I will say nothing against
the course of my existence.
But at bottom it has been
nothing but pain and
burden, and I can affirm
that during the whole of
my seventy-five years, I
have not had four weeks
of genuine well-being.

Johann Wolfgang von Goethe
1824

My external condition may
to many seem comfortable,
to some enviable but I think
that few men ever suffered
(in degree not in amount)
more genuine misery than I
have suffered.

Ralph Waldo Emerson
Journal, March 22, 1826

I frequently asked myself
if I could, or if I was bound
to go on living. . . . I generally answered to myself, that
I did not think I could pos-
sibly bear it beyond a year.

John Stuart Mill
Autobiography, *1873*

I am utterly weary of life.
I pray the Lord will come
forthwith and carry me
hence. Let him come, above
all, with his last
judgment: I will stretch out
my neck, the thunder will
burst forth, and I shall be at
rest. O God, grant that it
may come without delay.

Martin Luther

I have secluded myself
from society; and yet I
never meant any such
thing. . . . I have made a
captive of myself, and
put me into a dungeon
and now I cannot find
the key to let myself
out.

Nathaniel Hawthorne
Letter to Henry Wadsworth
Longfellow, June 1837

The Future
was a dark corridor
and at the far end
the door was bolted.

Gustave Flaubert
Madame Bovary, *1857*

The sky is darkening
like a stain,
Something is going to
fall like rain,
And it won't be flowers.

W. H. Auden
"The Witnesses"

The whole head is
sick, and the whole
heart faint.

Isaiah 1:5

Suicide is what the death certificate says when one dies of depression.

Peter D. Kramer, M.D.
The New York Times,
December 21, 1997

Everywhere
I see bliss,
from which I alone
am irrevocably
excluded.

Mary Wollstonecraft Shelley
Frankenstein, *1818*

Tears, idle tears, I know not
    what they mean,
Tears from the depth of
    some divine despair
Rise in the heart,
    and gather to the eyes.

Alfred, Lord Tennyson
"The Princess: A Medley," 1847

I got the
Weary Blues
And I can't be
satisfied.

Langston Hughes
The Weary Blues, *1926*

An intense feeling
carries with it its own
universe, magnificent
or wretched, as the
case may be.

Albert Camus
The Stranger, *1942*

I have
sometimes been
wildly, despairingly,
acutely miserable . . .

Dame Agatha Christie
An Autobiography, *1977*

I am the darkly shaded, the
bereaved, the disconsolate,
the prince of Aquitaine,
with the blasted tower.
My only star is dead, and
my star-strewn lute carries
on it the black sun of
melancholy.

Gérard de Nerval
El Desdichado *(The
Dispossessed), 1854*

Depression was a very active state really. Even if you appeared to an observer to be immobilized, your mind was in a frenzy of paralysis. You were unable to function, but were actively despising yourself for it.

Lisa Alther
Kinflicks, *1976*

To be *thoroughly*
conversant with a man's
heart, is to take our
final lesson in the
iron-clasped volume
of despair.

Edgar Allan Poe
Southern Literary Review,
June 1849

Despair is not an idea, it's a thing, a thing that tortures, squeezes, and breaks a man's heart. (Until he goes crazy and throws himself into the arms of death like the arms of a mother.)

Alfred-Victor, comte de Vigny
Chatterton, *1835*

Life is a well of joy, but for
those of whom
an upset stomach speaks
Which is the father of
melancholy
all wells are poisoned.

Friedrich Nietzsche
Thus Spake Zarathustra,
1883–91

Depression: 1. In the
normal individual, a state of
despondency characterized
by feeling of inadequacy,
lowered activity, and
pessimism about the future.
2. In pathological cases, an
extreme state of unrespon-
siveness to stimuli, together
with self-depreciation,
delusions of inadequacy,
and hopelessness.

J. P. Chaplin, Ph.D.
Dictionary of Psychology,
1975

The name of the
slough was
Despond.

John Bunyan
The Pilgrim's Progress, *1678*

From this slough of despond I try to raise myself by reading and re-reading Papa's speeches. . . . But I really cannot find the energy to read any serious work.

Sir Winston Churchill
Letter to his mother, 1895

I'm afraid the black dog
has really got me.
Churchill's image of despair
suits me better than "the
black hole." A black hole
just swallows you up.
Would that it were that
easy, to sink down into
darkness, as if sleeping.

Kathy Cronkite
On the Edge of Darkness,
1995

You handle
depression in much
the same way you
handle a tiger.

Dr. R. W. Shepherd
Quoted in Vogue *magazine,*
July 1978

Here rests his head
    upon the lap of Earth
A youth to Fortune and
    to Fame unknown,
Fair Science frown'd
    not on his humble birth,
And Melancholy mark'd
    him for her own.

Thomas Gray
"Elegy Written in a Country
Churchyard," 1751

Discomfort guides
my tongue
And bids me speak
of nothing but
despair.

William Shakespeare
The Comedy of Errors, *1595*

Woe
is wondrously
clinging: the
clouds ride by.

Anonymous

I want to be
forgotten even
by God.

Robert Browning

Let the day perish
wherein I was born,
and the night in which
it was said, There is a
man child conceived.

Job 3:30

Fly down,
   Death: Call me
I have become a
   lost name.

Muriel Rukeyser

There is much pain that is quite noiseless; and vibrations that make human agonies, are often a mere whisper in the roar of hurrying existence. There are glances of hatred that stab and raise no cry of murder; robberies that leave man or woman forever beggared of peace and joy, yet kept secret by the sufferer—committed to no sound except that made on the face by the slow months of suppressed anguish and early morning tears. Many an inherited sorrow that has marred a life has been breathed into no human ear.

George Eliot
Felix Holt, the Radical, *1866*

Believe me, every man
has his secret sorrows,
which the world
knows not;
and oftentimes we call
a man cold when he
is only sad.

Henry Wadsworth Longfellow
"The Light of Stars,"
Voices of the Night, *1839*

When a man has
lost all happiness
He's not alive. Call
him a breathing
corpse.

Sophocles
Antigone, *ca. 441* B.C.

Listen, Fred,
don't feel badly
when I die, because
I've been dead for a
long time.

Dorothy Parker

I been through
living for years.
I just ain't
dead yet.

Zora Neale Hurston
Moses: Man of the Mountain,
1939

I would
consent to
have a limb
amputated
to recover
my spirits.

Samuel Johnson

If a cloud knew
loneliness and fear,
I would be
that cloud.

Adrienne Rich

Loneliness and the
feeling of being
unwanted is the
most terrible poverty.

Mother Teresa

Someone call me
I can't stop crying
No one calls me
I feel like dying.

*Anonymous graffiti found
next to public telephone,
New York City, 1973*

There
have been
weeks
when no one
calls me
by
my name.

Leah Goldberg

I am in that temper
 that if I were under water
I would scarcely kick to
 come to the top.

John Keats

When water covers
the head, a hundred
fathoms are as one.

Persian proverb

Lately, I've become
accustomed to the way
the ground opens up
each time I go out to
walk the dog.

Amiri Baraka
(LeRoi Jones)

Ah, *mon cher*, for
anyone who is alone,
without God and
without a master, the
weight of days
is dreadful.

Albert Camus

I hear nothing, I speak nothing, I take interest in nothing, and from nothing to nothing I travel gently down the dull way which leads to becoming nothing.

Marie de Vichy-Chamrond,
Marquise du Deffand
Correspondence

Sadness is the
fundamental mood
of depression.

Julia Kristeva
Black Sun, *1987*

It isn't lightning, or
the beating of rain,
I'm simply sad, night
after night.

Tram Te Xuony
"Night Sadness"

A good woman feeling bad—that's the blues.

Anonymous

Je m'en vais enfin de ce monde, óu il faut que le coeur se brise ou se bronze.

And so I leave this world, where the heart must either break or turn to lead.

Sébastien-Roch Nicolas Chamfort
Suicide note, ca. 1794

Abody seriously out of equilibrium with itself or with its environment, perishes outright. Not so a mind. Madness and suffering can set themselves no limit.

George Santayana

When I was young, for two or three years the light faded out of the picture. I did not work. I sat in the House of Commons, but black depression settled on me. It helped me to talk to Clemmie about it. I don't like standing near the edge of a platform when an express train is passing through. I like to stand right back and if possible to get a pillar between me and the train. I don't like to stand by the side of a ship and look down into the water. A second's action would end everything. A few drops of desperation.

Sir Winston Churchill
August 14, 1944

A gloomy morning. On all sides a depressing outlook, and within, disgust with self.

Henri-Frédéric Amiel
Journal

Of all
the infirmities we
have,
the most savage
is to despise
our being.

Michel Eyquem de Montaigne

Is there no balm in
Gilead;
is there no physician
there?

Jeremiah 8:22

The main thing is
sadness . . . sorrow
is such that if I were
alone I would become
ill with grief.

Fyodor Dostoyevsky
Letter, May 27, 1869

Suffering
belongs to
no language.

Adélia Prado
The Alphabet in the Park:
Selected Poems of Adélia
Prado, *1990*

Despair is the worst
betrayal, the coldest
seduction: to believe at
last that the enemy
will prevail.

Marge Piercy
Reinventing Anarchy, *1979*

There is this difference
between depression and
sorrow—sorrowful, you are
in great trouble because
something matters so much;
depressed, you are miser-
able because nothing really
matters at all.

J. E. Buckrose
"Depression"
What I Have Gathered, *1923*

Real misery
cuts off all
paths to itself.

Dame Iris Murdoch
The Black Prince, *1973*

Who knows what loneliness is—not the conventional word but the naked terror?

Joseph Conrad

The grief that does
not speak
Whispers the
overfraught heart, and
bids it break.

William Shakespeare
Macbeth, *1606*

To fight aloud,
    is very brave—

But gallanter, I know

Who charge within
    the bosom

The Cavalry of Woe—

Emily Dickinson

Ah woe is me!
Winter is come
and gone.
But grief returns
with the revolving
year.

Percy Bysshe Shelley

Savrola dropped into
his chair. Yes, it had
been a long day, and a
gloomy day. . . . Was it
worth it?

Sir Winston Churchill
Savrola *(his only novel)*, *1900*

The flesh is sad,
alas, and I've read
all the books.

Stéphane Mallarmé
"Brise Marine"

Only one who is in pain
really senses nothing but himself;
pleasure does not enjoy itself but
something beside itself. Pain is
the only inner sense found by
introspection which can rival in
independence from experienced
objects the self-evident certainty
of logical and arithmetical
reasoning.

Hannah Arendt
Quoted in The Viking Book of
Aphorisms: A Personal Selection
by W. H. Auden and Louis
Kronenberger, 1962

Depression is . . . the antithesis of violence. It is a storm indeed, but a storm of murk. Soon evident are the slowed down responses, near paralysis, psychic energy throttled back close to zero. Ultimately the body is affected and feels sapped, drained.

William Styron
Darkness Visible, *1990*

The feeling
of Sunday is the
same everywhere,
heavy, melancholy,
standing still.

Jean Rhys
Voyage in the Dark, *1934*

I could not recall how much time had passed for somehow or other, pain is timeless, absolute. It has removed itself from space. It always has been and always will be, for it exists independent of relations.

Evelyn Scott

When you're
depressed there's no
calendar. There are
no dates, there's no day,
there's no night, there's
no seconds, there's
no minutes, there's
nothing. You're just
existing in this cold,
murky, ever-heavy
atmosphere.

Rod Steiger

Darkness and a troubled mind are a poor combination.

Frank L. Boyden
Quoted in Life *magazine,*
January 2, 1984

I have of late—but wherefore I know not—lost all my mirth, forgone all custom of exercise; and indeed it goes so heavily with my disposition, that this goodly frame, the earth, seems to me a sterile promontory; this most excellent canopy, the air, look you, this brave overhanging firmament, this majestical room fretted with golden fire, it appeareth nothing to me but a foul and pestilant congregation of vapors.

William Shakespeare
Hamlet, *1601*

Every day silence harvests its victims. Silence is a mortal illness.

Natalia Ginzburg
The Little Virtues, *1962*

Silence has
a suffocating,
deadening effect.
And the thing that
dies first is hope.

Katie Sherrod

Depression is caused by
the loss of hope.

Ronald Leifer
Quoted in Madness, Heresy, and
the Rumor of Angels *by Seth*
Farber and Thomas S. Szasz, 1993

I've already lost all hope.
I don't wait for joyful hours.
In fact night and day
  grieving,
I howl my agonies.
And as I suffer, I consume
Myself vilely and ask
  for death.

Kate Szidonis Petroczi

People commit suicide
for only one reason—
to escape torment.

Li Ang
The Butcher's Wife and Other
Stories, *1983*

"Then why these torments?" And the voice answered: "For no reason—they just are." Above and beyond this there was nothing.

Leo Tolstoy

Nobody comprehends
what a beast this
depression is. It has
stolen my life.

*A young woman speaking
about her illness, quoted in*
U.S. News & World
Report, *March 8, 1999*

Everything is
indifferent to me.
I *cannot* will
anything more;
often I do not know
whether I exist
or not.

Madame de Guion
1720

Melancholia: a
pathological state of
depression accompa-
nied by depressed
motor functions and
low reactivity to stimuli.

J. P. Chaplin, Ph.D.
Dictionary of Psychology,
1975

Like many people in personal turmoil, she rose late, didn't dress other than to cloak herself in her dressing gown, and she fell asleep easily through-out the day.

Carolyn Bly
"Talk of Heroes"

Day after day she
dragged her trouble
over to our house like a
sick animal she couldn't
cure, couldn't kill.

Margaret Millar
Beyond This Point
Are Monsters, *1970*

You come to realize that no matter how rich you are, there's no amount of money you can pay someone to fix you. There's no pill that's going to make you happy, no list of secret answers you can buy from the doctors, there's really nothing you can do except find it out for yourself.

Winona Ryder
Quoted in Parade *magazine,*
December 19, 1999

Suffering is
permanent and
obscure and dark
and shares the
nature of infinity—

William Wordsworth
The Borderers, *1842*

Me miserable! Which way shall I fly
Infinite wrath, and infinite despair?
Which way I fly is Hell, my self am Hell;
And in the lowest deep a lower deep
Still threatening to devour me opens wide,
To which the Hell I suffer seems a Heav'n.

John Milton
Paradise Lost, *1667*

I believe I am
in hell, therefore
I am there.

Arthur Rimbaud

What is hell?
Hell is oneself,
Hell is alone, the other figures in it
Merely projections. There is nothing to
    escape from
And nothing to escape to. One is always
    alone.

T. S. Eliot
The Cocktail Party, *1950*

Despair
is a greater deceiver than hope.

Luc de Vauvenargues
Reflections and Maxims,
1746

Pain hardens, and great pain hardens greatly, whatever the comforters say, and suffering does not ennoble, though it may occasionally lend a certain rigid dignity of manner to the suffering frame.

A. S. Byatt

In deep
sadness there is no
sentimentality.

William S. Burroughs

Whenever Richard Cory went downtown,
    We people on the pavement looked at him:
He was a gentleman from sole to crown,
    Clean favored, and imperially slim.

And he was always quietly arrayed,
    And he was always human when he talked;
But still he fluttered pulses when he said,
    "Good morning," and he glittered when he walked.

And he was rich—yes, richer than a king.
    And admirably schooled in every grace:
In fine, we thought that he was everything
    To make us wish that we were in his place.

So on we worked, and waited for the light,
    And went without the meat, and cursed the bread;
And Richard Cory, one calm summer night,
    Went home and put a bullet through his head.

Edwin Arlington Robinson
"Richard Cory,"
The Children of the Night, *1897*

April is the cruelest
   month, breeding
Lilacs out of the dead
   land, mixing
Memory and desire,
   stirring
Dull roots with
   spring rain.

T. S. Eliot
The Waste Land, *1922*

My life has been
brought to an impasse.
I loathe existence. . . .
Who am I? How did I
come into the world?

Søren Kierkegaard

Nobody knows
you. You are
the neighbor
of nothing.

Mark Strand

You are outside life, you are above life, you are afflicted with ills the ordinary person does not know, you transcend the normal level and that is what people hold against you, you poison their quietude, you corrode their stability. You feel repeated and fugitive pain, insoluble pain, pain outside thought, pain which is neither in the body, nor the mind, but which partakes of both.

Antonin Artaud

Something of glass about her,
   of dead water,
Chills and holds us,
Far more fatal than painted flesh
   or the lodestone of live hair
this despair of crystal brilliance.

Louis MacNeice
Poems, *1935*

She gives one the
impression that she is
now trapped in a pain
that is too old still to
cause tears.

Marguerite Duras
The Vice-Consul, *1965*

The happiness and unhappiness of men depend as much on their turn of mind as on fortune.

Duc François de La Rochefoucauld
Maxims, *1665*

Our happiness or
misery depends on our
dispositions, and not on
our circumstances.

Martha Washington

He who is of a calm
and happy nature will
hardly feel the pressure
of age, but to him who
is of an opposite dispo-
sition, youth and age
are equally a burden.

Plato
Republic, *fourth century* B.C.

Dying
Is an art, like
    everything else.
I do it exceptionally
    well.

Sylvia Plath
"Lady Lazarus," 1962

I was into pain
reduction and mind
expansion, but what
I've ended up with is
pain expansion and
mind reduction.

Carrie Fisher

Geez, if I could get
through to you, kiddo,
that depression is not
sobbing and crying and
giving vent, it is plain
and simple reduction of
feeling.

Judith Guest
Ordinary People, *1976*

Laugh and the world
laughs with you;
Weep and you weep
alone.

Ella Wheeler Wilcox
"Solitude,"
Poems of Passion, *1883*

There is a ladder
The ladder is always there
Hanging innocently
Close to the side of the
schooner.

Unattributed

The darkness and
the light are both
alike to thee.

Psalms 139:21

Yet from these flames
No light, but darkness
visible.

John Milton
Paradise Lost, *1667*

In the real dark
night of the soul it is
always three o'clock
in the morning.

F. Scott Fitzgerald

And I saw *darkness*
for weeks. It never
dawned on me that I
could come out of it.

Louise Nevelson
Dawns and Dusks, *1976*

Hello darkness, my
old friend
I've come to talk with
you again.

Paul Simon
"Sounds of Silence,"
Wednesday Morning, 3 AM,
1964

Warmth, warmth, more warmth! For we are dying of cold not of darkness. It is not the night that kills, but the frost.

Miguel de Unamuno
The Tragic Sense of Life in Men and Peoples, *1913*

Be near me when my light
  is low
When the blood creeps, and
The nerves prick
And tingle; and the heart is sick,
And all the wheels of Being
  slow.

Alfred, Lord Tennyson
In Memoriam, *1850*

The pain of the
mind is worse than
the pain of the body.

Publilius Syrus
First century B.C.

The black dog I hope always to resist, and in time to drive, though I am deprived of almost all those that used to help me. . . . When I rise my breakfast is solitary, the black dog waits to share it, from breakfast to dinner he continues barking, except that Dr. Brocklesby for a little keeps him at a distance. . . . Night comes at last, and some hours of restlessness and confusion bring me again to a day of solitude. What shall exclude the black dog from a habitation like this?

Samuel Johnson
Letter to Mrs. Thrale

Feel so low down an' sad, Lawd,
Feel so low down an' sad, Lawd,
Lost ev'rything I ever had.
Ain't got no friend nowhere, Lawd,
Ain't got no friend nowhere, Lawd,
All by myself no one to care.

Mercedes Gilbert
"Friendless Blues"

One who shows signs of mental aberration is, inevitably, perhaps, but cruelly shut off from familiar, thoughtless intercourse, partly excommunicated; his isolation is unwittingly proclaimed to him on every countenance by curiosity, indifference, aversion, or pity, and in so far as he is human enough to need free and equal communication and feel the lack of it, he suffers pain and loss of a kind and degree which others can only faintly imagine, and for the most part ignore.

Charles Horton Cooley
Human Nature and the Social Order,
1902

. . . because there is no escape from this smothering confinement, it is entirely natural that the victim begins to think ceaselessly of oblivion.

William Styron
Darkness Visible, *1990*

Ah, but to die and go we know
   not where
To lie in
Cold obstruction, and to rot.

William Shakespeare
Measure for Measure, *1604*

The Moon and Pleiades have set,
Midnight is nigh,
The time is passing, passing, yet
Alone I lie.

Sappho
Sixth century B.C.

Blue moon
You saw me standing alone
Without a song in my heart
Without a love of my own.

Richard Rogers and Lorenz Hart
"Blue Moon," ca. 1935

Joan her name was and
  at lunchtime
Solitary solitary
She would go and watch
  the pictures
In the National Gallery
All alone all alone
This time with no friend
  beside her
She would go and watch
  the pictures
All alone.

Stevie Smith

Beyond the curtain of
lianas, the rain falls
ceaselessly
Nostalgic atmosphere,
endless night
I seem to hear the
faint sound of footsteps
I am alone . . . unspeakable
misery.

Vu Hoang Chuong
"Nuages"

It is not good that
the man should
be alone.

Genesis 2:18

Then black despair,
the shadow
Of a starless night was
Thrown over the world
In which I moved alone.

Percy Bysshe Shelley
The Revolt of Islam, *1818*

There is no looking-glass here and I don't know what I am like now. I remember watching myself brush my hair and how my eyes looked back at me. The girl I saw was myself and yet not quite myself. Long ago when I was a child and very lonely I tried to kiss her. But the glass was between us— hard, cold and misted over with my breath. Now they have taken everything away. What am I doing in this place and who am I?

Mrs. Rochester speaking as a young girl in Jean Rhys's Wide Sargasso Sea, *1966, after she had been known for generations only as Mr. Rochester's mad wife in Emily Brontë's* Jane Eyre

What do I get—a couple of bucks and a one-way ticket to Palookaville. It was you, Charley. You was my brother. You should've looked out for me. Instead of making me take them dives for the short-end money. . . . You don't understand! I could've been a contender. I could've had class and been somebody. Real class. Instead of a bum, which I am.

Terry Malloy, played by Marlon Brando, to Charley Malloy, played by Rod Steiger, in Budd Schulberg's script for On the Waterfront, *1954*

Love, oh love,
  oh careless love,
All my happiness bereft,
You've filled my heart with
  weary old blues,
Now I'm talking to myself.

Spencer Williams and
Martha E. Koenig

I have heard the mermaids singing, each to each.
I do not think they will sing to me.

T. S. Eliot
"The Love Song of J. Alfred
Prufrock," 1915

But truly, I have wept too much! The Dawns are heartbreaking. Every moon is atrocious and every sun bitter.

Arthur Rimbaud
The Drunken Boat, *1871*

My soul is
a broken field
plowed by pain.

Sara Teasdale

It's funny when you feel as if you don't want anything more in your life except to sleep or else to lie without moving. That's when you can hear time sliding past you, like water running.

Jean Rhys
Voyage in the Dark, *1934*

Adieu tristesse
Bonjour tristesse
Tu es inscrite dans les
lignes du plafond.

Farewell sadness
Hello sadness
You are written in the lines
on the ceiling.

Paul Eluard
La Vie immédiate, *1932*

In the past men created witches; now they create mental patients.

Thomas S. Szasz

All that has to do with life is repugnant to me: everything that draws me to it horrifies me. I should like never to have been born, or to die. I have within me, deep within me, a distaste which keeps me from enjoying anything and which fills my soul to the point of suffocating it. It reappears in relation to everything, like the bloated bodies of dogs which come back to the surface of the water despite the stones that have been tied to their necks.

Gustave Flaubert
Correspondence

In the small hours
when the acrid stench
of existence rises like
sewer gas from every-
thing created, the
emptiness of my life
seems more terrible
than its misery.

Cyril Connolly

It seems my soul is
like a filthy pond,
wherein fish die
soon, and frogs
live long.

Thomas Fuller

He gnawed the rectitude of his life; he felt that he had been outcast from life's feast.

James Joyce
Ulysses, *1933 (written 1914–21)*

Sir Ralph the Rover
tore his hair;
He curst himself in his
despair.

Robert Southey
"The Inchcape Rock," ca. 1796

O God, O God,
How weary, stale, flat,
and unprofitable
Seem to me all the uses
of this world!

William Shakespeare
Hamlet, *1601*

Physical and social functioning are impaired by depression to a greater degree than by hypertension, diabetes, angina, arthritis, gastrointestinal diseases, lung problems or back ailments.

José Santiago, M.D.

Here I am, an old man in a
  dry month
Being read to by a boy, waiting
  for rain.

T. S. Eliot
"Gerontion," 1920

What makes
loneliness an
anguish is that
I have no one to
share my burden.

Dag Hammarskjöld

The lives of happy people are dense with their own doings—crowded, active, thick. . . . But the sorrowing are nomads, on a plain with few landmarks and no boundaries; sorrow's horizons are vague and its demands are few.

Larry McMurtry
Some Can Whistle, *1989*

Loneliness is the first
thing which God's eye
nam'd not good.

John Milton
Tetrachordon, *1644*

I do not need to go
out of my way to
express sadness and the
extreme of loneliness.

Vincent van Gogh
Letter to his brother,
Theo, 1890

What torments
my soul is
loneliness.

Eugène Delacroix

A lonely man is a lonesome thing, a stone, a bone, a stick, a receptacle for Gilbey's gin, a stooped figure sitting at the edge of a hotel bed, heaving copious sighs like the autumn wind.

John Cheever
Journal

I find the weight of air
Almost too great to bear.

Anne Morrow Lindbergh

About suffering they were
  never wrong.
The Old Masters: How well
  they understood
Its human position: how it
  takes place
While someone else is
  eating or opening a window
Or just walking along.

W. H. Auden
"Musée des Beaux Arts"

To be thoroughly con-
versant with a man's
heart is to take our final
lesson in the iron-
clasped volume of
despair.

Edgar Allan Poe
As editor of Southern Literary
Messenger, *1849*

My eyes
have only
one job:
to cry.

Nur Jahan

Frequent tears have run
the colors of my life.

Elizabeth Barrett Browning

. . . years dark with
torment and with tears.

Emily Brontë
"Sleep Not,"
Poems, *1846*

From childhood's hour
   I have not been
As others were—I have
   not seen
As others saw.

Edgar Allan Poe

When I was young, I said to Sorrow,
"Come and I will play with thee!"
He is near me all day
And at night returns to say
"I will come again tomorrow
I will come and stay with thee."

Aubrey Thomas De Vere
"When I Was Young, I Said to Sorrow"

At certain moments a single almost insignificant sorrow may, by association, bring together all the little relics of pain and discomfort, bodily and mental, that we have endured even from infancy.

Samuel Taylor Coleridge

Pain is real when you get
other people to believe in
it. If no one believes it but
you, your pain is madness
or hysteria.

Naomi Wolf
The Beauty Myth, *1990*

Men are never
convinced of your
reasons, of your
sincerity, of the
seriousness of your
sufferings, except by
your death.

Albert Camus
The Fall, *1956*

The obsession with
suicide is characteristic
of the man who can
neither live nor die, and
whose attention never
swerves from this
double impossibility.

E. M. Cioran
The New Gods

To be, or not to be; that is the question:
Whether 'tis nobler in the mind to suffer
The slings and arrows of outrageous
   fortune,
Or to take arms against a sea of troubles.
And by opposing, end them? To die:
   to sleep,
No more; and, by a sleep to say
   we end
The heartache.

William Shakespeare
Hamlet, *1601*

A still small voice
unto me
Thou art so full of
misery
Were it not better
not to be?

Alfred, Lord Tennyson
"The Two Voices," 1832

Whensoever any affliction assails me, me thinks I have the keys of my prison in mine owne hand, and no remedy presents it selfe so soone to my heart, as mine own sword.

John Donne
Biathanatos, *1644*

Let me get down on
the hearthrug, full of
laudanum
Grog, or as easy as may
be, into the nice wormy
grave.

Unattributed

I inherited a vile melancholy from my father which has made me mad.

Samuel Johnson

I am half mad from shadows, said the Lady of Chaillot.

Unattributed

It is a kind of
death to live in
wretchedness.

Ovid
The Poetic Epistles

Nobody heard him, the dead man,
But still he lay moaning:
I was much further out than you thought
And not waving but drowning.

Poor chap, he always loved larking
And now he's dead
It must have been too cold for him his
    heart gave way,
They said.

Oh, no no no, it was too cold always
(Still the dead one lay moaning)
I was much too far out all my life
And not waving but drowning.

Stevie Smith
"Not Waving but Drowning," 1957

We do not die of anguish, we live on. We continue to suffer. We drink the cup drop by drop.

George Sand
The Intimate Journal of
George Sand, *1929*

We are not miserable without feeling it. A ruined house is not miserable.

Blaise Pascal

The world leans on us. When we sag, the whole world seems to droop.

Eric Hoffer
Passionate State of Mind,
1955

I tell you naught for your comfort,
Yea, naught for your desire
Save that the sky grows darker yet
And the sea rises higher.

G. K. Chesterton
"The Ballad of the White Horse," 1911

Why so downcast my soul
Why do you sigh within me?

Psalms 42:5, 11

And it came to pass,
when the evil spirit from
God was upon Saul, that
David took up a harp
and played . . .
so Saul was refreshed,
and was well, and the evil
spirit departed from him.

1 Samuel 16:23

Nobody knows
what's in him until he
tries to pull it out.
If there's nothing or
very little, the shock
can kill a man.

Ernest Hemingway

I'm empty and aching and
I don't know why.
Counting the cars on the
New Jersey Turnpike. . .

Paul Simon
"America," 1964

As a painter I shall
never signify any-
thing of importance.
I feel it absolutely.

Vincent van Gogh

Yes, it is true that we
can have strawberries
in the spring—
but only for a short
time, and we are now
far from it.

Vincent van Gogh
Journal

It is hard to fight
an enemy who has
outposts in your
head.

Sally Kempton

Your mind now, moldering like
　wedding-cake,
heavy with useless experience,
　rich
with suspicion, rumour, fantasy,
crumbling to pieces under the
　knife-edge
of mere fact.　In the prime of
　your life.

Adrienne Rich
"Snapshots of a Daughter-in-Law,"
1987

The problems of alcoholism and drug addiction have strong links to depression. The search for highs may often begin as a flight from lows.

Nathan Kline, M.D.

The loneliness
persisted like
incessant rain.

Ann Allen Shockley
"Spring into Autumn"

A castle called
Doubting Castle, the
Owner whereof was
Giant Despair.

John Bunyan
The Pilgrim's Progress, *1678*

Melancholy and sadness are the start of doubt . . . doubt is the beginning of despair.

Comte de Lautréamont
(Isidore-Lucien Ducasse)
Poésies, *1870*

Despair . . . seeks
its own environment
as surely as water
finds its own level.

A. Alvarez

The country of
endured but unen-
durable pain.

Tennessee Williams
Quoted in The New York Times,
May 18, 1986

'Strange friend,' I said, 'here is no
   cause to mourn.'
'None,' said the other, 'save the
   undone years.
The hopelessness. Whatever hope is
   yours
Was my life also; I went hunting wild
After the wildest beauty in the world.'

Wilfred Owen
"Strange Meeting," 1917
(published posthumously, 1931)

To eat bread
without hope is still
to slowly starve
to death.

Pearl S. Buck
To My Daughters, with Love,
1967

. . . to have meat
and lack a stomach,
to lie in bed and
cannot rest.

William Camden

I cannot tell why this imagined
Despair has fallen upon me;
The ghost of an ancient legend
That will not let me be.

Heinrich Heine
"Lorelei"

Tired of the daily round
And tired of all my being
My ears are tired with sound
And mine eyes with seeing.

Mary Coleridge
1887

The lightening flashes through my skull; mine eyeballs ache and ache; my whole beaten brain seems as beheaded, and rolling on some stunning ground.

Herman Melville
Moby Dick, *1851*

My God, my God,
look upon me: why
hast thou forsaken
me?

Psalm 22

Being considered or labeled mentally disordered—abnormal, crazy, mad, psychotic, sick, it matters not what variant is used—is the most profoundly discrediting classification that can be imposed on a person today. Mental illness casts the "patient" out of our social order just as surely as heresy cast the "witch" out of medieval society.

Thomas S. Szasz in
The Manufacture of Madness: A Comparative Study of the Inquisition and the Mental Health Movement, *1970*

Cecily was not
likely to be cheerful,
and Cecily
depressed had the
art of clawing all the
emotional stuffing
out of people.

E. X. Ferrars
Cheat the Hangman, *1946*

She only said, 'My life is dreary,
He cometh not,' she said:
'I am aweary, aweary
I would that I were dead.'

Alfred, Lord Tennyson
"Mariana,"
Poems, Chiefly Lyrical, *1830*

Pain
has a
thousand
teeth.

Sir John William Watson
"The Dream of Man"

Death has a thousand doors to let out life, I shall find one. . . . From a loath'd life, I'll not an hour outlive.

Philip Massinger
A Very Woman, *ca. 1625*

Part of every misery is, so to speak, the misery's shadow or reflection: the fact that you don't merely suffer but have to keep on thinking about the fact that you suffer. I not only live each day in endless grief, but live each day thinking about living each day in grief.

C. S. Lewis
A Grief Observed

One of the depressing things about depression is knowing that there are lots of people in the world with far more reason to feel depressed than you have, and finding that, so far from making you snap out of your depression, it only makes you despise yourself more and thus feel more depressed.

David Lodge

Oh, if there is a man out of hell that suffers more than I do, I pity him!

Abraham Lincoln

Such incidents [of deafness, specifically when others were listening to music] drove me almost to despair. A little more of that and I would have ended my life—it was only my art that held me back.

Ludwig van Beethoven

There is no great
genius without some
touch of madness.

Seneca

Those whom God wishes to destroy, he first makes mad.

Euripides

We feel the machine slipping from
   our hands
As if someone else were steering.
If we see light at the end of the tunnel
It's the light of the oncoming train.

Robert Lowell
"Since 1939,"
Day by Day, *1977*

No worst, there
is none . . .
Comforter, where,
where is your
comforting?

Gerard Manley Hopkins
"No Worst, There Is None,"
1885

We work in the dark—we
do what we can—we give
what we have.

Henry James
"The Middle Years,"
Terminations, *1895*

I see my light come shining
From the west unto the east
Any day now, any day now
I shall be released.

Bob Dylan
"I Shall Be Released," 1967

I write of melancholy,
by being busy to avoid
being melancholy.

Robert Burton
The Anatomy of Melancholy, *1621*

In the river there is the crocodile. On the riverbank, there is the tiger. If you go to the forest, there are the thorns. If you go to the market, there is the policeman.

Anonymous

I long ago came to
the conclusion that
all life is six to five
against.

Damon Runyon
Money from Home, *1935*

Razors pain you;
Rivers are damp;
Acids stain you;
And drugs cause cramp.
Guns aren't lawful;
Nooses give;
Gas smells awful;
You might as well live.

Dorothy Parker
"Résumé," 1926

First I lost weight,
then I lost my voice,
and now I've lost
Onassis.

Maria Callas
1977

Nobody knows the
trouble you've seen—
and nobody wants to.

Helen Yglesias
Family Feeling, *1976*

A lover forsaken
A new love may get,
But a neck when
   once broken
Can never be set.

William Walsh

Now and then
there is a person born
who is so unlucky
that he runs into accidents
which started out to happen
to someone else.

Don Marquis
archys life of mehitabel, *1933*

It is always consoling to
think of suicide: in that
way one gets through
many a bad night.

Friedrich Nietzsche

There are few
sorrows, however
poignant, in which
a good income is of
no avail.

Logan Pearsall Smith

You may not know it, but at the far end of despair, there is a white clearing where one is almost happy.

Jean Anouilh

Life begins
on the other
side of despair.

Jean-Paul Sartre
The Flies, *1943*

If you have abandoned one faith, do not abandon all faith. There is always an alternative to the faith we lose.

Graham Greene
The Comedians, *1966*

When it is dark enough, you can see the stars.

Charles A. Beard

What does not
destroy me, makes
me strong.

Friedrich Nietzsche

Give us grace and strength to preserve. Give us courage and gaiety and the quiet mind. Spare to us our friends and soften to us our enemies. Give us the strength to encounter that which is to come, that we may be brave in peril, constant in tribulation, temperate in wrath and in all changes of fortune, and down to the gates of death, loyal and loving to one another.

Robert Louis Stevenson

In the depth of winter,
I finally learned that
within me there lay an
invincible summer.

Albert Camus

Sloppy,
raggedy-assed
old life.
I love it.
I never want
to die.

Dennis Trudell

Symptoms
of Depression

Depression has many levels: one can be mildly depressed, severely depressed, or anywhere in between. The symptoms, however, are relatively standard. If several or more of the following symptoms are present, you may be depressed and should seek help (see Resources).

• Loss of interest in life; boredom.

• Lack of energy and fatigue.

• Feelings of sadness or anxiety.

• Insomnia or excessive sleeping.

• Sense of isolation and loneliness.

• Feelings of guilt, worthlessness, or hopelessness.

• Major change in appetite or sudden loss or gain of weight.

• Loss of sex drive.

• Difficulty with memory, concentration, and decision making.

• Bouts of unexplained crying.

• Irritability, restlessness, thoughts of death or suicide.

• Various pains, such as headache or chest pain, without evidence of illness.

RESOURCES

If you believe that you are suffering from depression, please seek help. DO NOT WAIT. It is so difficult to find the right doctor, the right therapy and/or medication, but it must be done because you definitely can feel much better.

If you need immediate help, call 911, dial 0, or look in the front or back of your telephone book or on the Internet for local suicide hotlines. Unfortunately, there is no national 800 number that can direct you locally. It is, however, extremely important to talk to someone. Each of the fifty states has services to offer. Some, like New York and California, offer many resources; others, few. For example, if you're having a crisis anywhere in Georgia, you are referred to Gainsville, Florida. Some suggestions for telephone book or Internet searches include: Suicide Prevention, Samaritans, Crisis Center, and Mental Health. Stick with professionals and check credentials.

The following organizations can provide referrals to state and local affiliates for further information. Do not hesitate to contact them.

American Psychiatric Association
    1400 K St. NW
    Washington, D.C. 20005
    202-682-6000
    Web site: www.psych.org
    E-mail: apa@psych.org

Depression and Related Affective Disorders Association
  Meyer 3-181
  600 N. Wolfe St.
  Baltimore, MD 21287-7381
  410-955-4647 (Baltimore)
  202-955-5800 (Washington, D.C.)
  Web site: www.med.jhu.edu/drada/
  E-mail: drada@jhmi.edu

National Alliance for the Mentally Ill
  Colonial Place Three
  2107 Wilson Blvd., Ste. 300
  Arlington, VA 22201-3042
  1-800-950-6264
  Web site: www.nami.org

National Depressive and Manic Depressive Association
  730 N. Franklin St., Ste. 501
  Chicago, IL 60610-3526
  1-800-826-3632
  Web site: www.ndmda.org

National Institute of Mental Health
  6001 Executive Blvd., Room 8184, MSC 9663
  Bethesda, MD 20892-9663
  1-800-421-4311
  Web site: www.nimh.nih.gov
  E-mail: nimhinfo@nih.gov

National Mental Health Association
  1021 Prince St.
  Alexandria, VA 22314-2971
  1-800-969-6642
  Web site: www.nmha.org

BIOGRAPHICAL INDEX

Alther, Lisa (b. 1944). U.S. novelist. Best known for *Kinflicks*, a novel about coming of age in the 1960s, which critics compared favorably to the classic *Catcher in the Rye*.

Alvarez, A(lfred) (b. 1929). English critic and author. His poetry (*Apparition*) and fiction (*Hunt*) have been well received, but he has found most success as a critic. A leading advocate of "extremist" poets such as Robert Lowell and Anne Sexton.

Amiel, Henri-Frédéric (1821–1881). Swiss writer. Although a respected professor of aesthetics and philosophy, he considered himself a failure. His masterpiece is *Journal intime*, an introspective diary that he kept from 1847 until his death.

Ang, Li (b. ca. 1952). Chinese writer.

Anouilh, Jean (1910–1987). French playwright. Known for juxtaposing fantasy and reality, as in the dramas *Antigone* and *The Waltz of the Toreadors*.

Arendt, Hannah (1906–1975). U.S. (German-born) writer, political philosopher, and educator. Her work *The Origins of Totalitarianism* established her as a major political thinker. Her other works include *The Human Condition*, *Eichmann in Jerusalem*, and *The Life of the Mind*.

Artaud, Antonin (1896–1948). French actor, critic, and drama theorist. A Surrealist and originator of the Theater of Cruelty movement, he focused on dreams and the mind's interior workings.

Auden, W(ystan) H(ugh) (1907–1973). U.S. (English-born) poet and critic. His collections include *The Dance of Death* and *The Double Man*.

Baraka, Amiri (b. 1934). Born LeRoi Jones. U.S. dramatist and political activist. Best known for his plays *The Slave* and *Dutchman*, which deal with racism and the African-American experience. Changed his name after converting to Islam in 1967, but has since adopted a Marxist philosophy.

Beard, Charles A. (1874–1948). U.S. historian. Author of *An Economic Interpretation of the Constitution of the United States*. Resigned from Columbia University in 1917 over the issue of academic freedom during wartime.

Beethoven, Ludwig van (1770–1827). German composer. Often considered the greatest of all composers. Despite losing his hearing by 1798 and becoming completely deaf in 1819, his works include nine symphonies, twenty sets of piano variations, and seventeen string quartets.

Blake, William (1757–1827). English poet and artist. His paintings and poetic works have a mystical, visionary quality, as in the poetry collection *Songs of Innocence* and the prophetic book *The Marriage of Heaven and Hell*.

Bly, Carolyn (b. 1930). U.S. writer. Explores the essence of small-town life in her short-story collection *Backbone* and in the essay collection *Letters from the Country*.

Boyden, Frank L. (1879–1972). Former headmaster, the Deerfield Academy, Deerfield, Massachusetts.

Brontë, Emily (1818–1848). English poet and novelist. Sister to novelists Charlotte and Anne. A former governess, she is best known for *Wuthering Heights*, her only novel, and is today considered one of the foremost poets of her time.

Browning, Elizabeth Barrett (1806–1861). English poet. Her first poems were published at age nineteen. Best known for the love sonnets she wrote to her husband, the poet Robert Browning, with whom she eloped despite her ill health and her father's disapproval.

Browning, Robert (1812–1889). English poet. Husband of the poet Elizabeth Barrett Browning. Best known for the four-volume collection *The Ring and the Book* and his dramatic monologues, including "My Last Duchess" and "The Bishop Orders His Tomb."

Buck, Pearl S. (1892–1973). U.S. writer. Well known for her novels about life in China, where she was raised by her missionary parents until 1934. Received the 1932 Pulitzer Prize and the 1938 Nobel Prize for literature. Her novel *East Wind: West Wind* addressed the issue of the bound feet of Chinese women, and *The Good Earth* described farm life in China.

Buckrose, J. E. (1868–1931). Pseudonym of Annie Edith Foster. English writer.

Bunyan, John (1628–1688). English preacher and writer. Celebrated for *The Pilgrim's Progress*, the allegorical tale of the hero Christian's journey from the City of Destruction to the Celestial City.

Burroughs, William S. (1914–1997). U.S. writer. Best known for his novel *Naked Lunch*, which helped establish him as a figure of the Beat movement. He wrote of his experiences as a heroin addict in *Junkie*.

Burton, Robert (1577–1640). English clergyman. Author of *The Anatomy of Melancholy*, which went beyond the causes and cures of melancholy to paint a picture of contemporary life and outline a plan for utopia.

Byatt, A(ntonia) S(usan) (b. 1936). English writer. Sister of the writer Margaret Drabble. Creator of complex, sophisticated novels and short stories. Best known for the novel *Possession*, which received the Booker Prize in 1990.

Callas, Maria (1923–1977). Greek-U.S. coloratura soprano. Well known for her intensity. Among her notable roles was

Bellini's *Norma*. Made her European debut in 1947 and her U.S. debut in 1956.

Camden, William (1551–1623). English antiquarian and historian. He compiled *Britannia*, a pioneering topographical survey of the English Isles.

Camus, Albert (1913–1960). French writer and philosopher. His works concern the absurdity of the human condition, as in *The Stranger* and *The Plague*. Received the Nobel Prize for literature in 1957. Died in an automobile accident.

Chamfort, Sébastien-Roch Nicolas (1741–ca. 1794). French author, Jacobin revolutionary, and wit. Sources do not agree on whether he was killed on orders from the French Convention or whether he committed suicide.

Chaplin, J. P., Ph.D. U.S. author. Wrote the *Dictionary of Psychology*.

Cheever, John (1912–1982). U.S. writer. His short stories and novels depicted life in America's suburbs with humor and compassion. Received the Pulitzer Prize in 1979 for *The Stories of John Cheever*.

Chesterton, G. K. (1874–1936). English writer and critic. Known for his Father Brown detective novels and volumes of criticism.

Christie, Dame Agatha (1890–1976). English writer. Author of more than seventy detective novels, including *And Then There Were None* and *The Murder of Roger Ackroyd*.

Churchill, Sir Winston (1874–1965). English politician and writer. As prime minister, he inspired European resistance to Germany as he led Great Britain through World War II. Author of numerous histories and biographies, he received the 1953 Nobel Prize for literature.

Cioran, Emil (1911–1995). French (Romanian-born) philosopher and writer. His contributions to French-language prose made him a foremost writer in the mid- to late twentieth century. His works include *Of Tears and Saints* and *A Short History of Decay*.

Coleridge, Mary (1861–1907). English poet. Great-great-niece of Samuel Taylor Coleridge. Best known for her novel *The King with Two Faces*, but more attention is now being paid to her lyrical poetry, as in the collection *Fancy's Following*.

Coleridge, Samuel Taylor (1772–1834). English poet and critic. Published, with William Wordsworth, *Lyrical Ballads*, which contains "The Rime of the Ancient Mariner," his best-known poem. After breaking with Wordsworth, he published "Christabel" and "Kubla Khan."

Connolly, Cyril (1903–1974). English author and literary critic. A journalist for the London *Sunday Times* who also wrote essays and a novel, *The Rock Pool*.

Conrad, Joseph (1857–1924). English (Ukrainian-born to Polish parents) novelist. His works include *Lord Jim* and *Heart of Darkness*. A master of creating emotionally isolated characters suffering from loss of moral integrity.

Cooley, Charles Horton (1864–1929). U.S. sociologist. Developed the theory that the human mind is social by nature and that society is a mental construct.

Cronkite, Kathy (b. ca. 1952). U.S. writer and actress. Her works include *On the Edge of Darkness*, a collection of interviews with famous figures who have conquered depression.

Deffand, Marie de Vichy-Chamrond, Marquise du (1697–1780). French writer and hostess. Established the brilliant salon that attracted intellectuals and aristocrats. Known for her witty, acerbic writings and her correspondence with the writers Voltaire and Horace Walpole.

Delacroix, Eugène (1798–1863). French painter and leader of the Romantic movement. Known for his huge, dramatic canvases and exuberant use of color, as in *Liberty Leading the People* and *The Massacre at Chios*.

de Nerval, Gérard (1808–1855). Pseudonym of Gérard Labrunie. French Symbolist poet and translator. Died by his own hand a year after completing *Aurélia*, an account of his journey to understand the demons that assailed his mind and soul.

de Unamuno, Miguel (1864–1936). Spanish author and philosopher. Writer of mystical philosophy, poetry, and historical studies. Best known for the philosophical work *The Tragic Sense of Life in Men and Peoples*.

De Vere, Aubrey Thomas (1814–1902). Irish poet and critic. Wrote devotional verse and hymns in strong, lyrical, spiritual language.

Dickinson, Emily Elizabeth (1830–1886). U.S. poet. Virtually a recluse at her home in Amherst, Massachusetts, she wrote more than a thousand poems of great depth and elegance.

Donne, John (1572–1631). English metaphysical poet and clergyman. He served as chaplain to James I and was dean of Saint Paul's Cathedral in London from 1621 until his death. His works include *Divine Poems* and the prose work *Biathanatos*, published posthumously. Known for his brilliant use of paradox, hyperbole, and imagery.

Dostoyevsky, Fyodor (1821–1881). Russian writer. His works reflect both his insight and his mysticism. His most important novels are *Crime and Punishment* and *The Brothers Karamazov*.

Duras, Marguerite (b. 1914). French (Vietnamese-born) author and Marxist. Author of the screenplay *Hiroshima, Mon Amour* and the autobiographical novel *The Lover*.

Dylan, Bob (b. 1941). Born Robert Zimmerman. U.S. song-writer. His revolutionary song "Blowin' in the Wind" became an anthem of the civil rights movement in the 1960s. His albums *Highway 61 Revisited* and *Blonde on Blonde* revolutionized rock music.

Eliot, George (1819–1880). Pseudonym of Mary Ann Evans. English writer. Her moralistic novels include *Adam Bede*, *Silas Marner*, and her masterpiece, *Middlemarch*.

Eliot, T(homas) S(tearns) (1888–1965). English (U.S.-born) critic and writer. Known for his provocative, unconventional poems, including "The Love Song of J. Alfred Prufrock" and "The Waste Land," and his dramas, including *Murder in the Cathedral* and *The Cocktail Party*. Received the 1948 Nobel Prize for literature.

Eluard, Paul (1895–1952). French poet. A founder of the Surrealist movement in literature. Coined the phrase *bonjour tristesse* (hello sadness), which became the title of Françoise Sagan's best-selling 1950s novel.

Emerson, Ralph Waldo (1803–1882). U.S. writer, philosopher, and transcendentalist. His poems, prose, and essays, such as the book *Nature*, were landmarks in the development of U.S. liter-ary thought and expression.

Euripides (ca. 480–406 B.C.). Greek poet and dramatist. Considered one of the greatest of classical tragedians, along with Sophocles and Aeschylus. Author of *Medea*, *Hippolytus*, and *The Trojan Women*, he focused on less-than-heroic characters.

Ferrars, E. X. (1907–1995). Pseudonym of Morna Doris Brown, also known as Elizabeth Ferrars. English (Burmese-born) author. Popular and prolific writer of detective fiction. Her mysteries include *Kill or Cure* and *Cheat the Hangman*.

Fisher, Carrie (b. 1956). U.S. actress and writer. A featured actress in the *Star Wars* trilogy, she later emerged as a success-

THE LITTLE BOOK OF HOPE

ful novelist and screenwriter. Her novels include *Postcards from the Edge* and *Delusions of Grandma*.

Fitzgerald, F(rancis) Scott (Key) (1896–1940). U.S. writer. One of the most memorable figures of the jazz age along with his wife, Zelda, also a writer, and others, including Ernest Hemingway. His best-known and still widely read novels are *The Great Gatsby* and *Tender Is the Night*.

Fitzgerald, Zelda Sayre (1900–1948). U.S. writer. Wife of the writer F. Scott Fitzgerald. Her works include *Save Me the Waltz*. Died eight years after her husband, when a fire consumed the asylum in which she was undergoing treatment for mental illness.

Flaubert, Gustave (1821–1880). French writer. Admired for his precise style and realistic novels, among them *Madame Bovary*, *Salammbô*, and *A Sentimental Education*.

Freud, Sigmund (1856–1939). Austrian psychiatrist and founder of psychoanalysis. His psychoanalytic theories, which initially were met with disbelief and hostility, later profoundly influenced many areas of twentieth-century thought.

Frost, Robert (1874–1963). U.S. poet. His works, widely read and usually set in rural New England, often explore the relationship between humankind and nature. His collections include *A Boy's Will* and *In the Clearing*.

Fry, Stephen (b. 1957). English actor and writer. A frequent performer on stage, screen, and television, he has published the novel *The Liar*, the autobiographical *Moab Is My Washpot*, and *Fry and Laurie 4* (written with Hugh Laurie).

Fuller, Thomas (1608–1661). English clergyman. Author of several important historical works known for their wit and puns, including *The Church History of Britain*.

Gilbert, Mercedes (1889–1952). U.S. actress, songwriter, and novelist. One of the few black women of her time to both act and write, she appeared in Langston Hughes's play *Mulatto*. The songs "Decatur Street Blues" and "Got the World in a Jug" were set to her poems. Her plays and novels include *Environment* and *Aunt Sara's Wooden God*.

Ginzburg, Natalia (1916–1991). Italian writer. One of the best-known postwar Italian writers, her intimate, authentic explorations of domestic life include *A Life for Fools* and *Voices in the Evening*.

Goethe, Johann Wolfgang von (1749–1832). German writer and scientist. Best known for his dramatic poem *Faust*, in which a magician and alchemist sells his soul to the devil. In his scientific work he combined sensuous experience with poetic intuition.

Goldberg, Leah (1911–1970). Israeli (Lithuanian-born) poet, critic, and educator. One of the most respected lyrical poets of Israel, she was influenced by both Western and Eastern European Symbolists. Her poetry collections include *Rings of Smoke*.

Gray, Thomas (1716–1771). English poet and forerunner of English Romanticism. His most famous work is "Elegy Written in a Country Churchyard."

Greene, Graham (1904–1991). English writer. Most admired for his intense, moralistic novels, which include *The End of the Affair* and *The Power and the Glory*. He also wrote the script for the 1950 film classic *The Third Man*.

Guest, Judith (b. 1936). U.S. novelist. Best known for the novel *Ordinary People*, which was made into an Academy Award–winning film.

Hammarskjöld, Dag (1905–1961). Swedish diplomat. As Secretary-General of the United Nations from 1953 to 1961, he helped settle differences between nations related to the Cold War and those that arose from the struggle for independence by African nations. Died in a plane crash while on a mission to the Congo (now Zaire).

THE LITTLE BOOK OF HOPE

Hawthorne, Nathaniel (1804–1864). U.S. writer. Best known for his moralistic, elegantly written novels, including *The Scarlet Letter* and *The House of the Seven Gables*. Helped establish the U.S. short story as an art form.

Heine, Heinrich (1797–1856). German poet and essayist. Published the poetry collection *Pictures of Travel*. His revolutionary opinions made it difficult for him to find work in Germany. He went to Paris after 1830, where he turned to politics.

Hemingway, Ernest (1899–1961). U.S. writer and journalist. His novels are considered unparalleled in their rendering of courage and loneliness, as in *The Sun Also Rises*, *For Whom the Bell Tolls*, and *The Old Man and the Sea*. Received the Nobel Prize for literature in 1954. Died by his own hand.

Hoffer, Eric (1902–1983). U.S. longshoreman and philosopher. Wrote of life and the soul in such works as *The True Believer*.

Hopkins, Gerard Manley (1844–1889). English poet and cleric. Known for a number of works published posthumously, including "The Wreck of the Deutschland" and "The Windhover."

Hughes, Langston (1902–1967). U.S. writer. Best known for his poetry collection *The Weary Blues* and his story collection *The Ways of White Folks*. His poetry, prose, and drama were important contributions to the Harlem Renaissance.

Hugo, Victor (1802–1885). French writer. Exiled in 1851 after Napoléon III came to power, he returned to France in 1870. His great novels include *The Hunchback of Notre Dame* and *Les Misérables*.

Hurston, Zora Neale (1903–1960). U.S. writer and folklorist. She celebrated the African-American folklore of the rural South in her novels *Their Eyes Were Watching God* and *Moses: Man of the Mountain* and was a key contributor to the Harlem Renaissance.

James, Henry (1843–1916). English (U.S.-born) writer and critic. His works generally concern the clash between U.S. and European cultures. Author of numerous psychological novels, including *The Bostonians* and *The Golden Bowl*.

Johnson, Samuel (1709–1784). English writer and lexicographer. Known as Dr. Johnson, he was England's leading literary figure in the second half of the eighteenth century.

Joyce, James (1882–1941). Irish writer. A master of language whose literary innovations greatly influenced modern fiction. His masterpiece is *Ulysses*, completed in 1921 but not published in the United States until 1933 due to obscenity charges. Also wrote *Dubliners* and *Finnegans Wake*.

Keats, John (1795–1821). English poet. Considered one of the greatest poets of the English language. His works, melodic and rich in classical imagery, include "The Eve of St. Agnes," "Ode on a Grecian Urn," and "To Autumn."

Kempton, Sally (b. 1943). U.S. writer.

Kierkegaard, Søren (1813–1855). Danish theologian and philosopher. A forerunner of existentialism, he insisted on the need for individual decision and leaps of faith. His works include *Either/Or* and *Fear and Trembling*.

Kingsolver, Barbara (b. 1955). U.S. writer. Her works, often set in the U.S. Southwest, include the novels *Animal Dreams*, *The Bean Trees*, and *The Poisonwood Bible*.

Kramer, Peter D., M.D. (b. 1948). U.S. psychiatrist and writer. Author of the best-selling *Listening to Prozac: A Psychiatrist Explores Anti-Depressant Drugs and the Remaking of the Self*.

Kristeva, Julia (b. 1941). French (Bulgarian-born) author, philosopher, and psychoanalyst. Her works, which include *Powers of Horror* and *Black Sun*, focus on language, literature, and cultural history.

Lansdowne, first marquis of (1737–1805). Born William Petty. English politician. Opposed the Stamp Act as secretary of state and later helped negotiate the Treaty of Paris.

La Rochefoucauld, François, duc de (1613–1680). French classical writer. Penned wise and witty aphorisms, published as *Maxims*. His pessimistic view of human selfishness helped earn him a place in French literature.

Lautréamont, comte de (1846–1870). Pseudonym of Isidore-Lucien Ducasse. French (Uruguayan-born) poet. Enigmatic figure in French literature who was held up by the Surrealists as an exemplar. Wrote the prose epic *Les Chants de Maldoror*.

Lewis, C(live) S(taples) (1898–1963). English academic, writer, and critic. Most famous for his series of children's books, *The Chronicles of Narnia*. His autobiography, *Surprised by Joy*, was written after his conversion to Christianity.

Lincoln, Abraham (1809–1865). Sixteenth president of the United States (1861–65). He brilliantly and courageously led the Union during the Civil War and emancipated the slaves in the South. Assassinated shortly after the end of the war by actor and Southern sympathizer John Wilkes Booth.

Lindbergh, Anne Morrow (b. 1906). U.S. aviator and writer. Wife of aviator Charles Lindbergh, whom she accompanied on many of his flights. Author of *North to the Orient* and *Listen! the Wind*.

Lodge, David (b. 1935). English novelist and critic. His works include *Language of Fiction*, *The Novelist at the Crossroads*, and *After Bakhtin*.

Longfellow, Henry Wadsworth (1807–1882). U.S. writer and poet. His works include the narrative poem "Song of Hiawatha" and a translation of Dante's *Divine Comedy*.

Lowell, Robert (1917–1977). U.S. poet. His works include the confessional *Life Studies* and the autobiographical *Land of Unlikeness*. Received the Pulitzer Prize in 1947 for *Lord Weary's Castle*.

Luther, Martin (1483–1546). German theologian and leader of the Protestant Reformation. Prompted by the corruption and abuse he saw on the part of papal emissaries in Rome, he wrote and posted his historic Ninety-five Theses, which angered the Church and led to his excommunication. He later established the Lutheran Church.

MacNeice, Louis (1907–1963). English (Irish-born) poet. His works treat social issues in a detached, often ironic manner, as in *Blind Fireworks* and other collections.

Mallarmé, Stéphane (1842–1898). French Symbolist poet. Believed poetry should be abstract and transcendental. His works include *The Afternoon of a Faun*, translated by Edgar Allan Poe.

Marquis, Don (1878–1937). U.S. poet, novelist, and humorist. Creator of the popular archy and mehitabel stories, which chronicle the adventures of a cockroach (archy) and an alley cat (mehitabel).

Massinger, Philip (1583–1640). English playwright of satirical comedies. Harsh moralist best known for the satire *A New Way to Pay Old Debts*. Many of his plays are lost.

McMurtry, Larry (b. 1936). U.S. novelist. Best known for his Southwestern themes, as in the trilogy consisting of *The Last Picture Show*, *Texasville*, and *Dwayne's Depressed*. Received the 1986 Pulitzer Prize for the novel *Lonesome Dove*.

Melville, Herman (1819–1891). U.S. writer. His masterpiece, *Moby Dick*, is considered one of the greatest novels in the English language.

Mill, John Stuart (1806–1873). English philosopher and economist. Best known for his interpretations of empiricism and utilitarianism.

Millar, Margaret (1915–1944). U.S. (Canadian-born) writer. Wife of Kenneth Millar, aka Ross Macdonald. Author of numerous noteworthy mysteries. Received the Edgar award for *A Beast in View* in 1955.

Milton, John (1608–1674). English poet and scholar. Best known for the epic poem *Paradise Lost*, an account of humanity's fall from grace, which he wrote in retirement following the English Restoration. It is considered by many to be the finest epic in the English language.

Montaigne, Michel Eyquem de (1533–1592). French essayist and politician. Mayor of Bordeaux (1581–1585), he introduced the essay as a literary genre.

Murdoch, Dame Iris (1919–1999). English (Irish-born) writer. Her complex, philosophical novels include *Under the Net* and *The Sea, the Sea*.

Nevelson, Louise (1900–1988). U.S. (Russian-born) sculptor. Her massive, abstract "environmental" works, including huge walls of stacked, boxlike shapes, were often created from cast metal, wood, and found objects.

Nietzsche, Friedrich (1844–1900). German philosopher. He reasoned that Christianity's emphasis on the afterlife made its believers less able to cope with earthly life. Author of *Beyond Good and Evil* and *Thus Spake Zarathustra*.

Nightingale, Florence (1820–1910). English (Italian-born) nurse and hospital reformer. Known as the Lady of the Lamp. Considered the founder of modern nursing, she organized and directed a unit of field nurses during the Crimean War and helped improve conditions for the war-wounded.

264

Norris, Kathleen (1880–1966). U.S. novelist. Author of *Bread into Roses* and *Barberry Bush*.

Nur Jahan ("Light of the World") (1571–1645). Born Mihr-un-Nisa. Poet and empress of India. Wife of the emperor Jahangir (ruled 1605–27). She was a strong political influence on her husband and set new fashion trends based on Persian traditions.

Ovid (43 B.C.–A.D. 17). Roman poet. Best known for his explorations of love, as in *The Art of Love* and *Metamorphoses*.

Owen, Wilfred (1893–1918). English poet. His works reflect the horror and cruelty he saw during World War I. Died in battle a week before the Armistice. Most of his poems were published posthumously.

Parker, Dorothy (1893–1967). U.S. writer. Drama critic for *Vanity Fair*, book critic for the *New Yorker*, and author of numerous short stories and poems. Best known for her satirical wit.

Pascal, Blaise (1623–1662). French philosopher and mathematician. He developed the modern theory of probability and discovered the properties of cycloids. His experiments led to the invention of the hydraulic press.

Piercy, Marge (b. 1936). U.S. writer. Her politically charged, often documentary-style novels include *Small Changes* and *Woman on the Edge of Time*.

Plath, Sylvia (1932–1963). U.S. writer. Best known for her poems, filled with images of alienation, as in her collections *The Colossus and Ariel*, and her novel *The Bell Jar*. Died by her own hand.

Plato (ca. 427–347 B.C.). Greek philosopher. Student of Socrates, teacher of Aristotle, and founder of the Academy in Athens. Considered the most important figure in Western philosophy. Best known for his theory that ideal Forms or Ideas, such as Truth or Good, exist in a realm beyond the material world.

Poe, Edgar Allan (1809–1849). U.S. writer. Best known for his dark poems such as "The Raven," and his macabre short stories, including "The Fall of the House of Usher" and "The Tell-Tale Heart."

Prado, Adélia (b. 1936). Brazilian writer and poet. She explores Brazilian life and spiritual relationships from a feminine perspective, as in the poetry collection *Luggage*.

Publilius Syrus (first century B.C.). Roman writer. Best known for his versified maxims taken from his dialogues by later scholars.

Rhys, Jean (1894–1979). Pseudonym of Gwen Williams. English (West Indian–born) writer. Best known for *Wide Sargasso Sea*, a novel whose main character is the young Mrs. Rochester from Charlotte Brontë's classic *Jane Eyre*.

Rich, Adrienne (b. 1929). U.S. poet, author, and feminist. *Dark Fields of the Republic: Poems 1991–1995* is among her collections. Her nonfiction prose includes *Of Woman Born*.

Rimbaud, Arthur (1854–1891). French poet. His dreamlike works, including the collection *Illuminations*, influenced the Symbolists. After *A Season in Hell* received a chilly reception, he quit writing at age nineteen and spent the rest of his life wandering through Europe and Africa.

Robinson, Edwin Arlington (1869–1935). U.S. poet. Best known for his short, dramatic, revelatory poems, such as "Miniver Cheevy" and "Richard Cory," set in a fictional New England town. Received Pulitzer Prizes in 1922, 1925, and 1928.

Rukeyser, Muriel (1913–1980). U.S. writer. Her feminist poetry speaks out against racism and war, as in *The Gates: Poems* and *Beast in View*. She believed poetry has the power to encourage humankind to realize its fullest potential.

Runyon, Damon (1884–1946). U.S. writer. Best known for his humorous, slangy insider stories about Broadway and the New York underworld, as in *Guys and Dolls*.

Ryder, Winona (b. 1971). U.S. actress. Intense, versatile performer whose films include *Bram Stoker's Dracula*, *The Age of Innocence*, and *Girl, Interrupted*.

Saint-Exupéry, Antoine de (1900–1944). French writer and aviator. Best known for his fairy tale for adults, *The Little Prince*. Lost in action during World War II.

Sand, George (1804–1876). Pseudonym of Amandine Dupin, Baroness Dudevant. French writer. Her works, which include more than 100 books, concern the independence of women, as in *Valentine* and *Consuelo*. She is also known for her love affairs with the composer Frédéric Chopin and the writer Jules Sandeau, among others.

Santayana, George (1863–1952). U.S. (Spanish-born) philosopher and writer. Best known for his theories of aesthetics, morality, and the spiritual life. In addition to his philosophical works, such as the four-volume *Realms of Being*, he wrote poetry and a novel, *The Last Puritan*.

Sappho (flourished ca. 610–580 B.C.). Greek lyric poet. Although only fragments of her simple but passionate lyrics survive, she is considered an important literary voice and the greatest of the early Greek lyric poets.

Sarton, May (1912–1995). U.S. (Belgian-born) poet and novelist. The key theme of her works is the nature and benefits of solitude. Published the poetry collections *Inner Landscape* and *A Private Mythology*.

Sartre, Jean-Paul (1905–1980). French writer and existential philosopher. His works include the play *No Exit* and the philosophical treatise *Being and Nothingness*. He declined the 1964 Nobel Prize for literature.

Schulberg, Budd (b. 1914). U.S. novelist and screenwriter. Best known for his screenplay *On the Waterfront* and for his best-selling novel *What Makes Sammy Run?*, which shocked Hollywood with its hard-hitting depiction of people in the film industry.

Scott, Evelyn (1893–1963). U.S. writer and poet. Her first autobiography, *Escapade*, focused on her shifting psychological states while living in poverty in Brazil. Published the novel *Eva Gay* and the poetry collection *Precipitations*.

Seneca (ca. 4 B.C.–A.D. 65). Roman Stoic philosopher, writer, orator, and tutor of Nero. Son of Seneca the Elder. His works influenced Renaissance and Elizabethan drama. Died by his own hand.

Sexton, Anne (1928–1974). U.S. poet. Her works document her struggle with mental illness and her search for faith, as in the collections *Live or Die* and *The Death Notebooks*. Died by her own hand.

Shakespeare, William (1564–1616). English poet and dramatist. His body of work—including numerous sonnets, tragedies such as *Hamlet* and *King Lear*, historical plays such as *Richard II*, and comedies such as *As You Like It* and *Much Ado about Nothing*—is considered among the most important in English literature.

Shelley, Mary Wollstonecraft (1797–1851). English writer. Wife of the poet Percy Bysshe Shelley. Best known for the gothic novel *Frankenstein*.

Shelley, Percy Bysshe (1792–1822). English Romanticist poet. Husband of the writer Mary Wollstonecraft Shelley. His works include the lyrics "Ode to the West Wind," the verse drama *Prometheus Unbound*, and *Adonais*, an elegy to the poet John Keats.

Sherrod, Katie. U.S. writer.

Shockley, Ann Allen (b. 1927). U.S. writer and educator. *Loving Her* and *Say Jesus and Come to Me*, which explore lesbian love, are among her novels. Her provocative works focus on women's issues and racism against African Americans.

Simon, Paul (b. 1941). U.S. songwriter and poet. Best known for the albums *Sounds of Silence* and *Bridge over Troubled Water* (both with Art Garfunkel), *Graceland*, and *Rhythm of the Saints*.

Smith, Logan Pearsall (1865–1946). English (U.S.-born) author and essayist. Best known for his essay collections and his short stories.

Smith, Stevie (1902–1971). Pseudonym of Florence Margaret Smith. English poet. Her collected poems—including *A Good Time Was Had by All*—are still in print, her witty but sad voice still popular.

Sophocles (ca. 496–406 B.C.). Greek tragic poet and dramatist. Considered one of the greatest dramatists of ancient Greece, along with Euripides and Aeschylus. His innovations profoundly influenced Western tragedy. His surviving plays include *Ajax*, *Oedipus Rex*, *Antigone*, and *Oedipus at Colonus*.

Southey, Robert (1774–1843). English writer. Once a political radical, he is best known for his Romantic poetry, biographical works, and criticism, as well as his friendship with the poets Coleridge and Wordsworth.

Steiger, Rod (b. 1925). U.S. actor. An intense Method actor, he starred in *The Pawnbroker*, *On the Waterfront*, and *In the Heat of the Night*, receiving an Academy Award for the latter.

Stevenson, Robert Louis (1850–1894). Scottish writer. His works include the adventure classic *Treasure Island* and the moralistic thriller *The Strange Case of Dr. Jekyll and Mr. Hyde*. A tuberculosis sufferer, he eventually settled in Samoa, where he died, leaving two unfinished works.

Strand, Mark (b. 1934). U.S. (Canadian-born) poet and poet laureate (1990–91). His collections include *Sleeping with One Eye Open*, *Reasons for Moving*, *Darker*, and *Blizzard of One*. Received the 1999 Pulitzer Prize.

Styron, William B. (b. 1925). U.S. writer. Best known for his powerful novels, which include *Lie Down in Darkness* and *Sophie's Choice*. His autobiographical book on depression, *Darkness Visible*, is considered one of the best lay books on the subject.

Szasz, Thomas S. (b. 1920). U.S. (Hungarian-born) psychiatrist. His books espouse that all disease is physical, and that "mental disease" is thus a myth. He believes all human behavior is purposeful and intentional.

Teasdale, Sara (1884–1933). U.S. poet. Her lyrical works have appeared in *Love Songs* (for which she received the 1917 Pulitzer Prize) and other collections. Died by her own hand.

Tennyson, Alfred, first baron (1809–1892). Known as Alfred, Lord Tennyson. English poet and poet laureate (1850–92). His works reflect both Victorian feelings and aesthetics, as in *In Memoriam* and "The Charge of the Light Brigade."

Teresa, Mother (1910–1997). Born Agnes Gonxha Bojaxhiu to Albanian parents in Skopje (now Macedonia). Roman Catholic missionary. Devoted her life to relieving the suffering of India's impoverished and desperate people. Founder of the Missionaries of Charity. Received the 1979 Nobel Peace Prize.

Tolstoy, Count Leo (1828–1910). Born Lev Nikolayevich Tolstoy. Russian writer and philosopher. His two greatest novels, *War and Peace* and *Anna Karenina*, are filled with unusually vivid detail and extraordinary psychological insight.

Tram Te Xuony. Vietnamese poet.

Trudell, Dennis. U.S. poet. His works uncover the hope and humor in the world's grim reality and emphasize the connection between all people on earth. Published the collections *Fragments of Us* and *The Guest*.

van Gogh, Vincent (1853–1890). Dutch Postimpressionist painter. His works include numerous self-portraits, a vivid series of sunflower paintings, and the famous *Starry Night*. Died by his own hand.

Vauvenargues, Luc de Clapiers de, Marquis (1715–1747). French soldier and moralist. Sought heroic fulfillment by enlisting in the army. Anticipated Rousseau's and Stendhal's views of humankind with his *Reflections and Maxims*.

Vigny, Alfred-Victor, comte de (1797–1863). French author and translator. A Romantic writer, his works include the historical novel *Cinq-Mars* and the play *Chatterton*.

Vu, Hoang Chuong (1916–1976). Vietnamese poet. A member of the Au Lac people of Vietnam, his rich, lyrical works include "Home Longings."

Walsh, William (1916–1996). English educator and writer. His writings include *A Human Idiom* and *Coleridge: The Work and the Relevance*.

Washington, Martha (1731–1802). U.S. hostess and patriot. George Washington was her second husband. She was the first U.S. woman to be depicted on a U.S. postage stamp.

Watson, Sir John William (1858–1935). English poet and author. Wrote political and lyrical verse and sonnets. *The Prince's Quest* and *Wordsworth's Grave* are among his better-known works.

Wilcox, Ella Wheeler (1850–1919). U.S. journalist and poet. Completed her first novel at the age of ten. Author of the narrative poem *Maurine* and the collection *Poems of Passion*.

Williams, Spencer (ca. 1889–1965), and **Koenig, Martha E.** U.S. songwriters. Williams's songs, which remain popular today, include "I Ain't Got Nobody," "Basin Street Blues," and "Squeeze Me," the latter cowritten with Fats Waller.

Williams, Tennessee (1911–1983). U.S. playwright. His dramas, full of human passion and frustration, include *A Streetcar Named Desire* and *Cat on a Hot Tin Roof*. He also wrote short stories and novels.

Wolf, Naomi (b. 1962). U.S. writer and feminist. Her works include *The Beauty Myth* and *Promiscuities*. She is a frequent lecturer on women's issues.

Wordsworth, William (1770–1850). English poet and poet laureate (1843). His most important collection, *Lyrical Ballads*, cowritten with the poet Samuel Taylor Coleridge, helped introduce Romanticism to England.

Yglesias, Helen (b. 1915). U.S. writer. A former literary editor, her rich, intelligent novels, such as *How She Died*, *Family Feeling*, and *Sweetsir*, focus on the position of women in urban society.